are you My Mother?

A NICU infant's journey in search of her mother

By Lori Brecto

Illustrated by Penny Weber

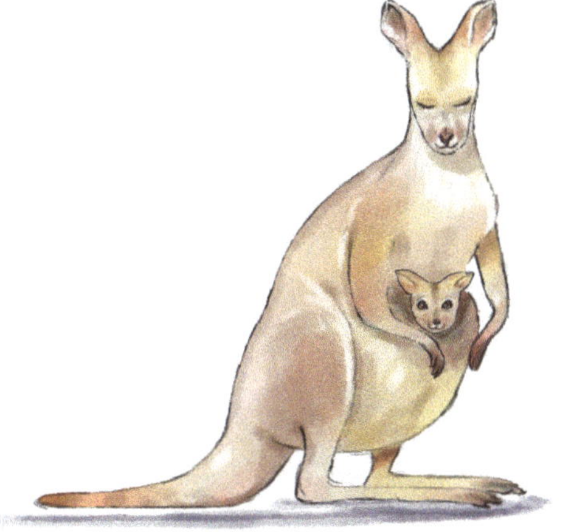

Copyright © 2024 by Lori Brecto
Illustrations by Penny Weber
Creative Design: Linda H. Powers / PowersDesign.net

All rights reserved. No portion of this book may be reproduced in any form without permission from the author, except as permitted by U.S. copyright law.

ISBN 979-8-218-39810-1 Hardcover
ISBN 979-8-218-39811-8 Paperback

For permissions contact: Lori Brecto / brectoes@yahoo.com

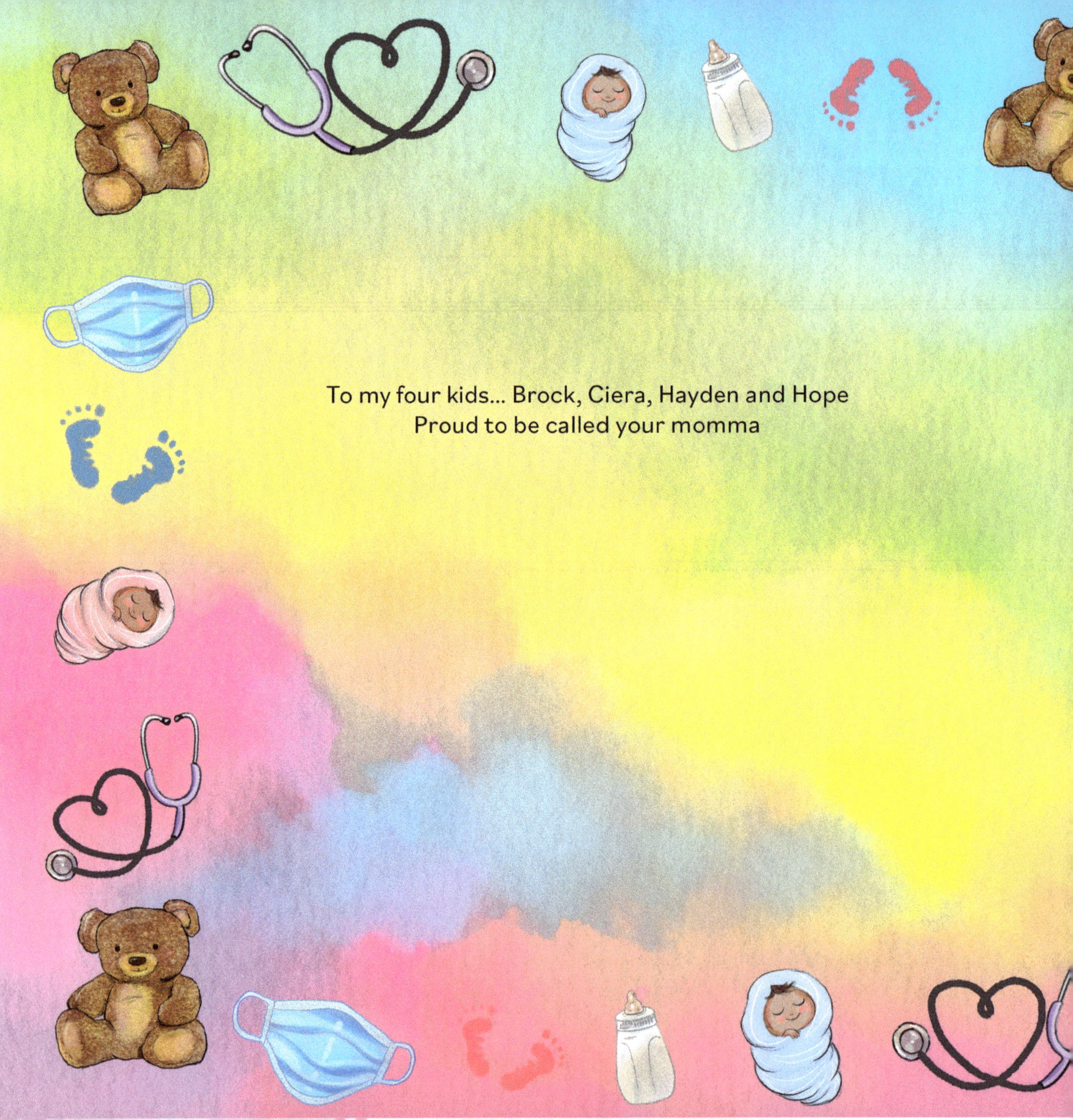

To my four kids... Brock, Ciera, Hayden and Hope
Proud to be called your momma

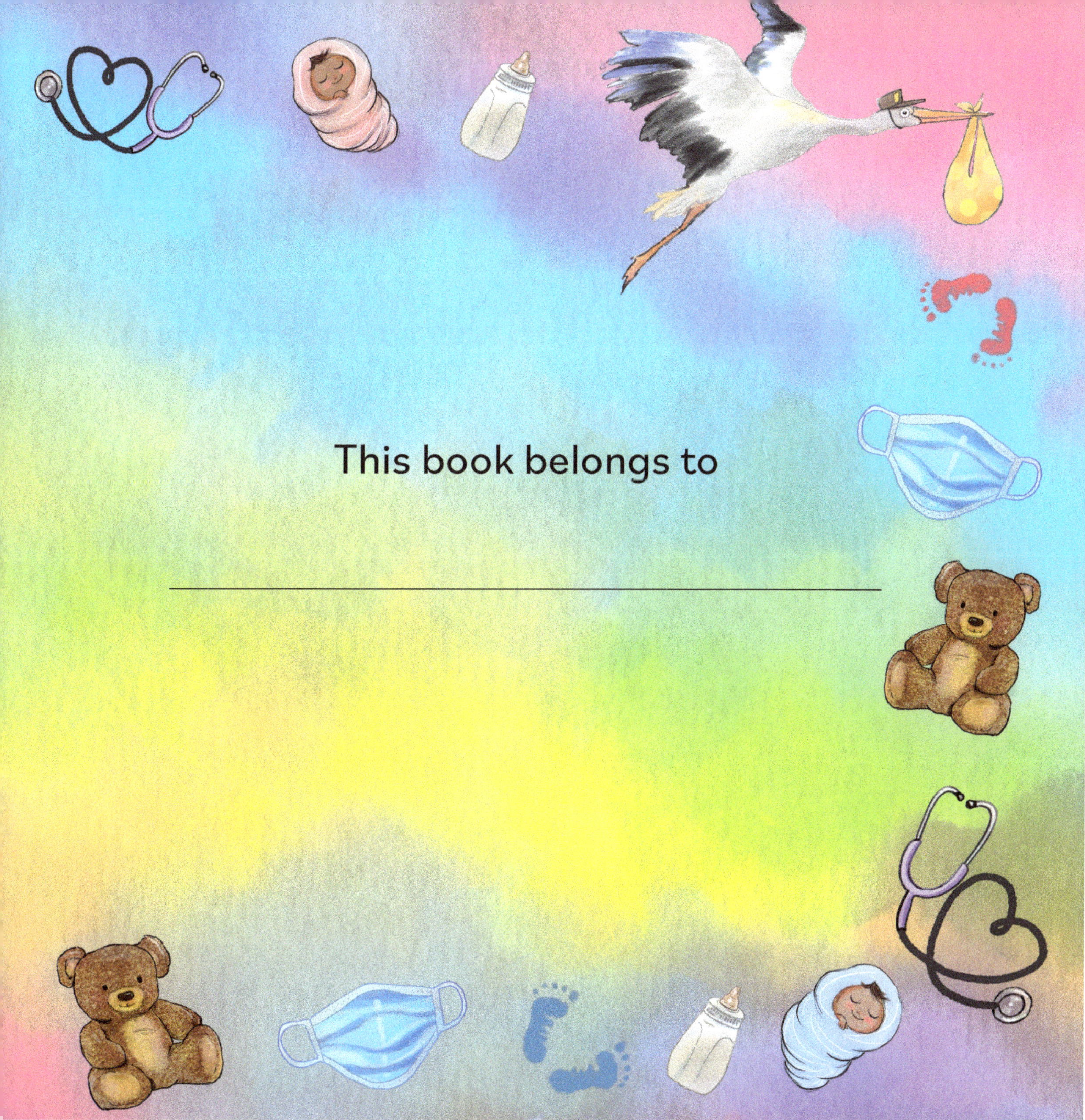
This book belongs to

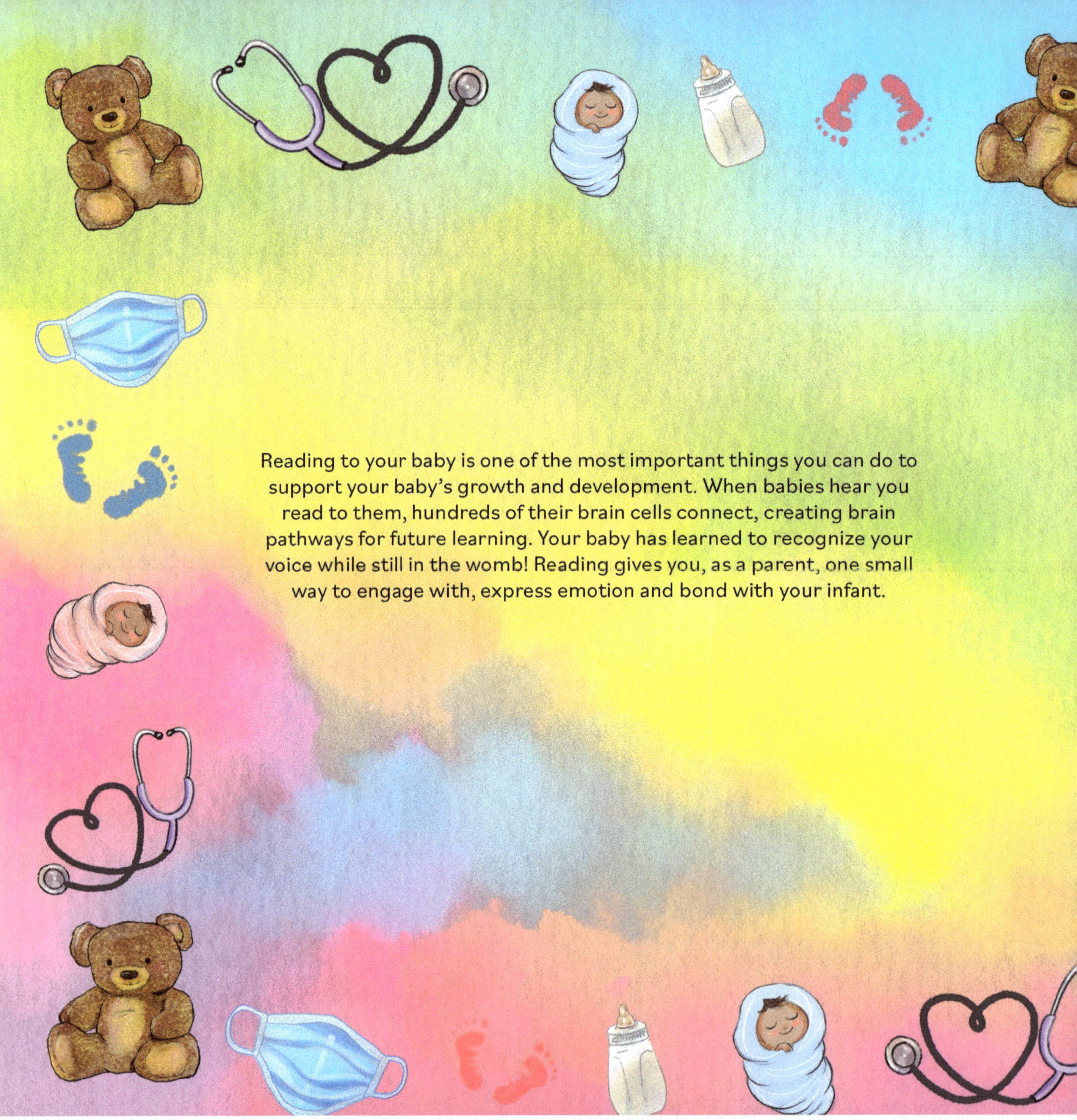

Reading to your baby is one of the most important things you can do to support your baby's growth and development. When babies hear you read to them, hundreds of their brain cells connect, creating brain pathways for future learning. Your baby has learned to recognize your voice while still in the womb! Reading gives you, as a parent, one small way to engage with, express emotion and bond with your infant.

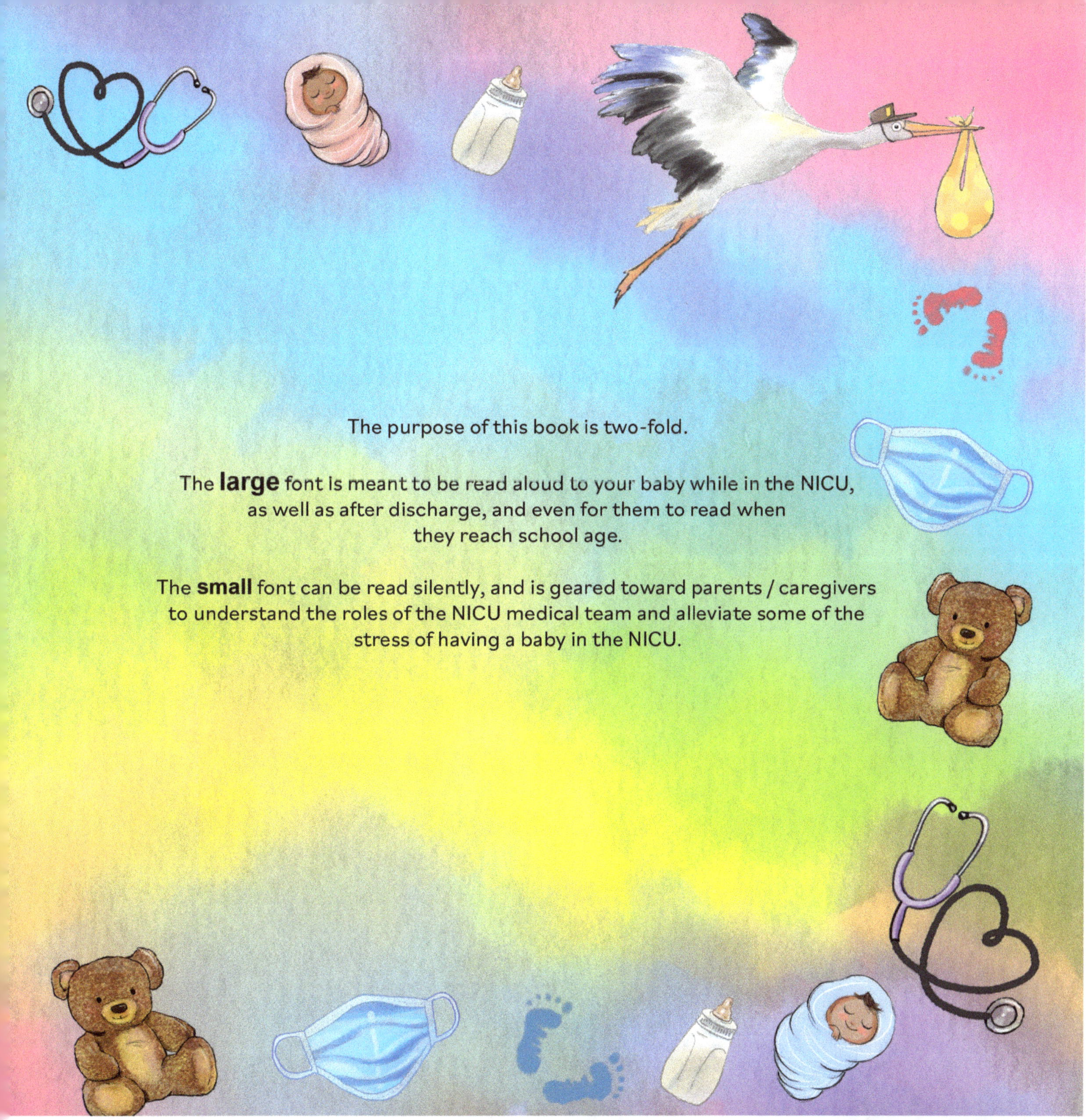

The purpose of this book is two-fold.

The **large** font is meant to be read aloud to your baby while in the NICU, as well as after discharge, and even for them to read when they reach school age.

The **small** font can be read silently, and is geared toward parents / caregivers to understand the roles of the NICU medical team and alleviate some of the stress of having a baby in the NICU.

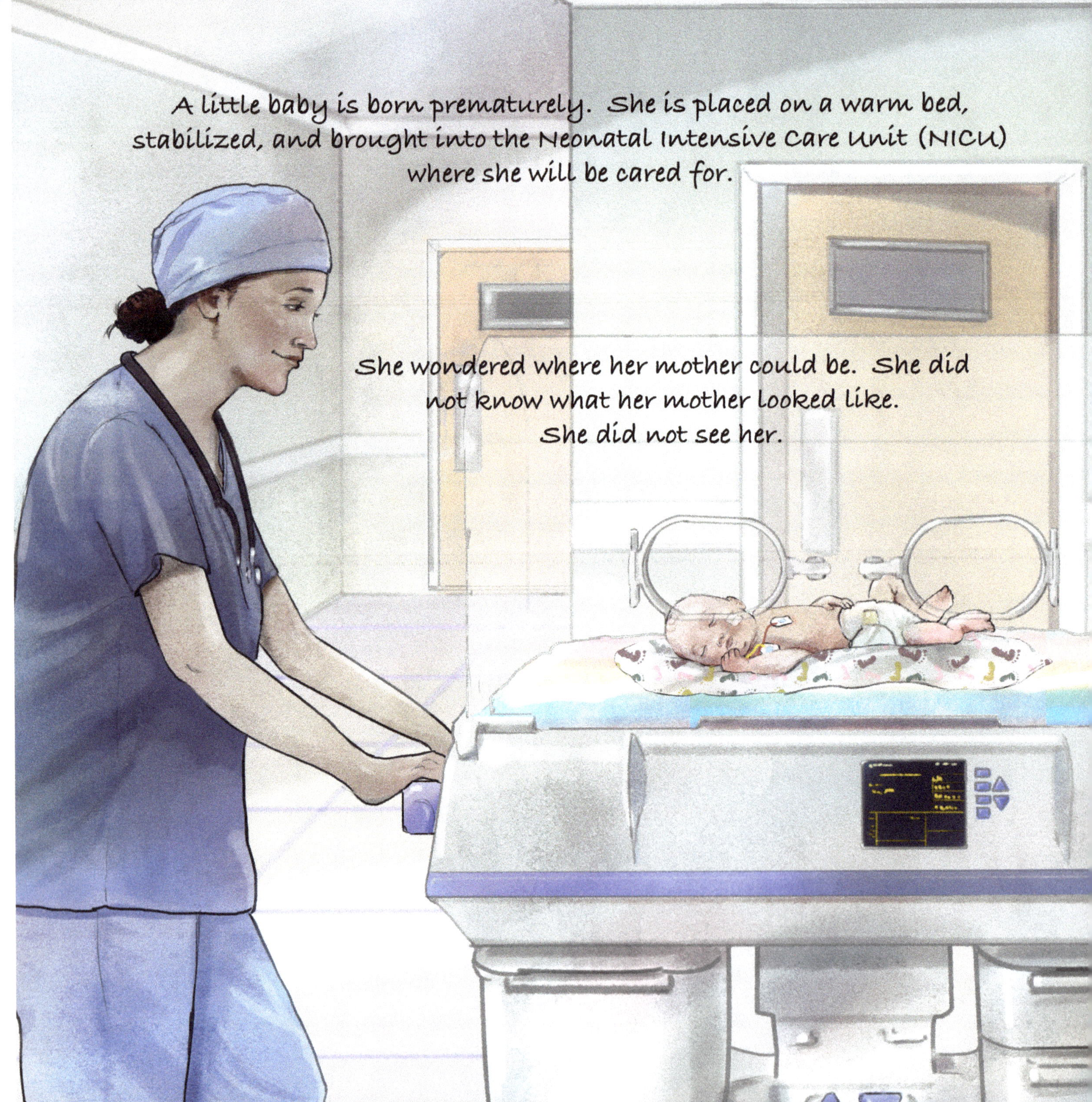

A little baby is born prematurely. She is placed on a warm bed, stabilized, and brought into the Neonatal Intensive Care Unit (NICU) where she will be cared for.
She wondered where her mother could be. She did not know what her mother looked like.
She did not see her.

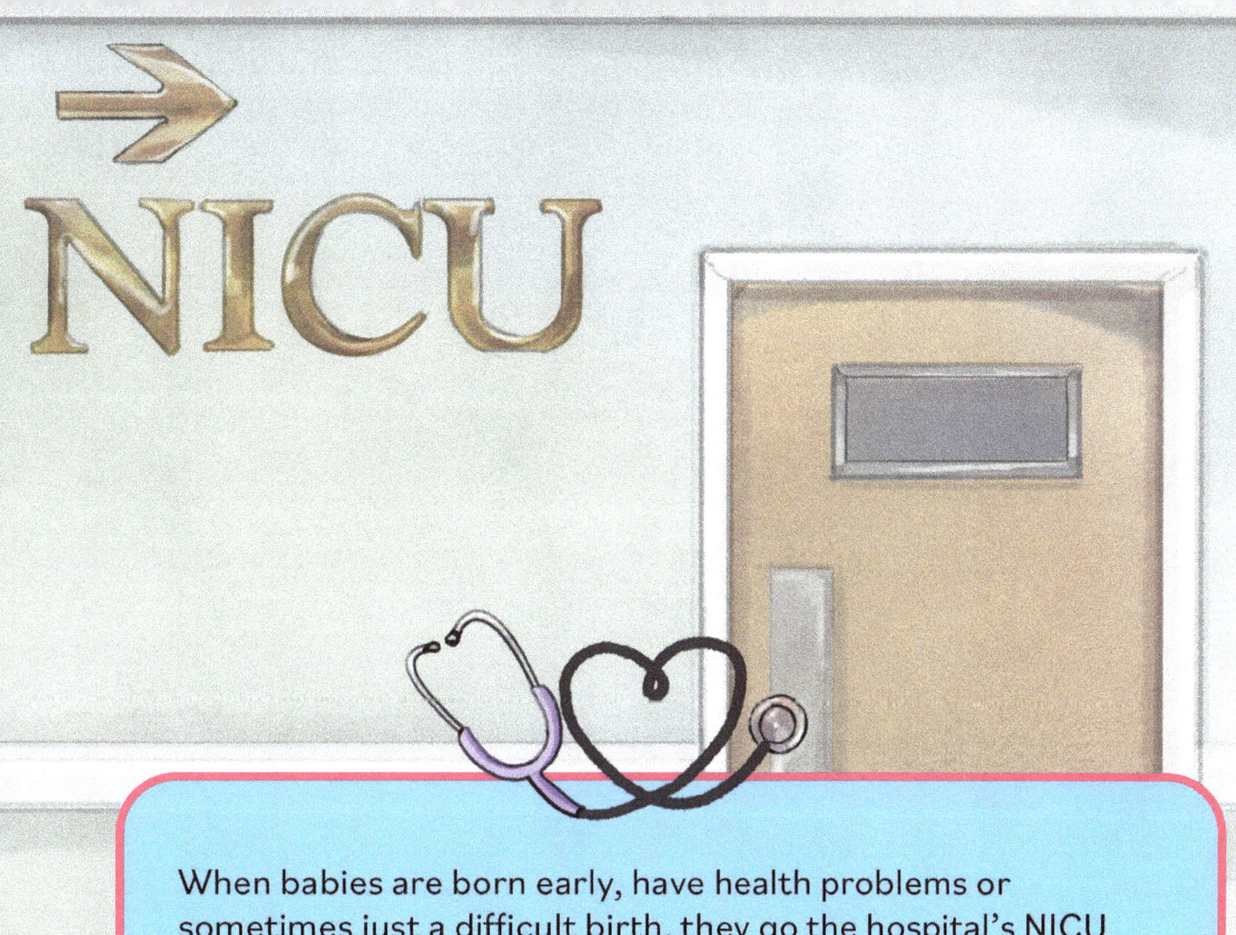

When babies are born early, have health problems or sometimes just a difficult birth, they go the hospital's NICU.

NICU stands for Neonatal Intensive Care Unit. While there, your baby will be provided around the clock care.

There will be health care providers who have special training and equipment to give your baby the best possible care. In the U.S., 1 out of 10 babies is born prematurely.

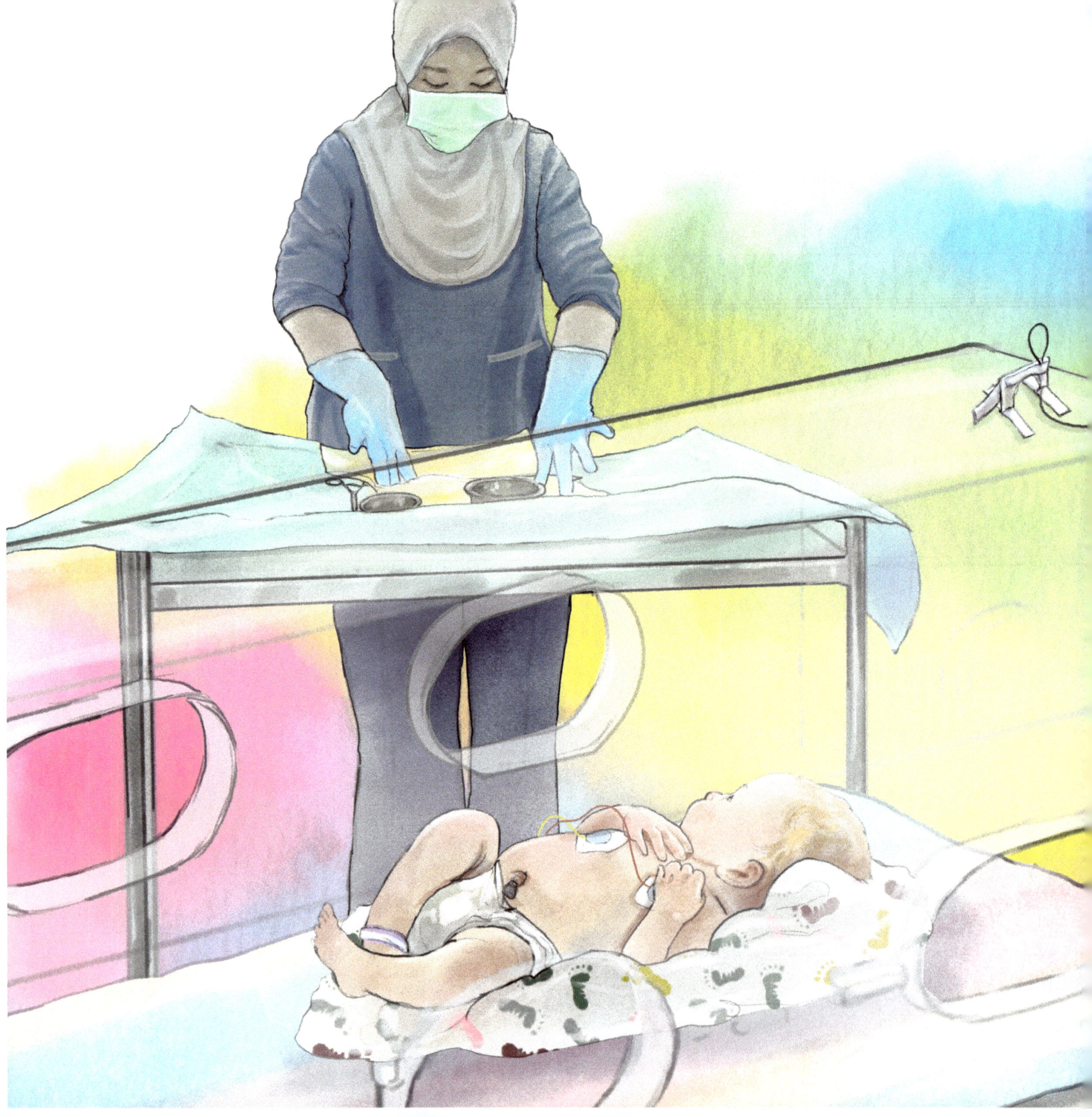

"Where is my mother?", she thought.

The baby saw someone with a face mask and cap, wearing
a paper gown, preparing to place a catheter that would
provide fluid and nutrition.

"Are you my mother?" she asked.
"No, little one. I am the Neonatal Nurse Practitioner",
said the NNP.

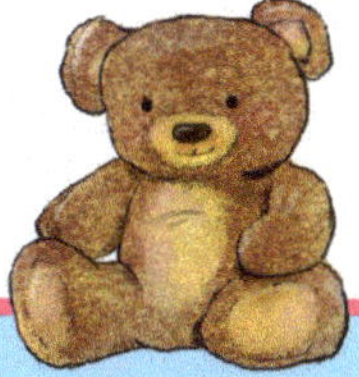

A **Neonatal Nurse Practioner** (NNP) is a registered nurse with
specialized training in caring for high risk infants who need care due
to low birth weight, prematurity, infections or other conditions.

An NNP works closely with the neonatologist to diagnose and treat
illness and provide the best possible care for your baby.

You may meet many different NNPs from the medical team
throughout your baby's stay.

The baby looked around and saw someone setting
up a ventilator.

"Are you my mother?" she asked.

The respiratory therapist just
continued with his work.
He did not say a thing.

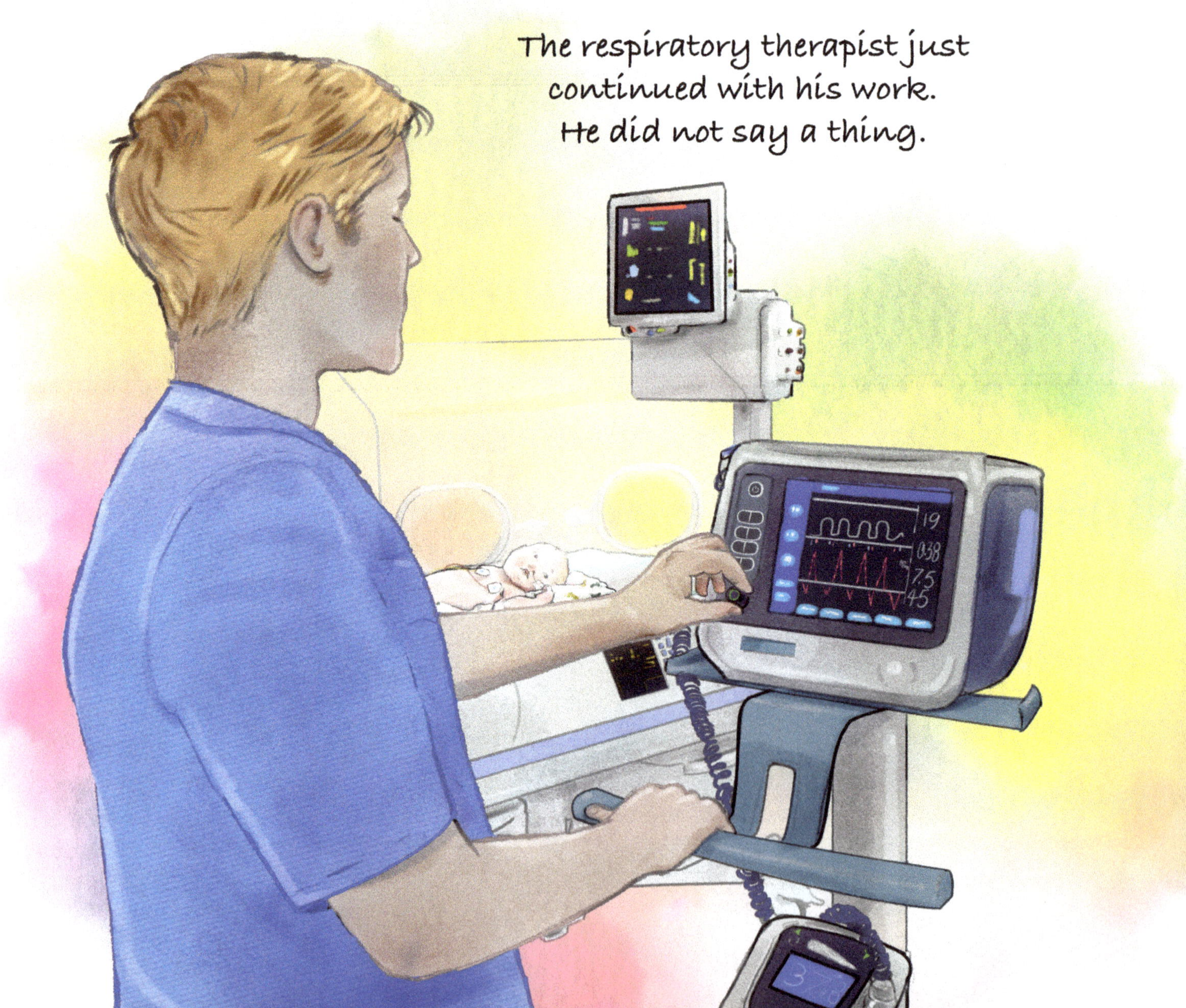

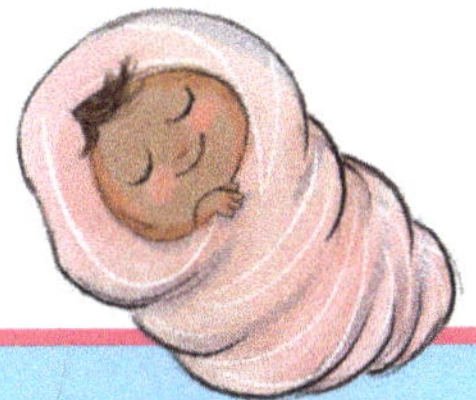

A large percentage of babies in the NICU will initially experience respiratory distress. **Respiratory Therapists** (RTs) are specifically trained to assess, care for, and monitor babies with breathing difficulties to ensure they get the support they need.

This may include monitoring placement of breathing tubes, managing ventilators and breathing masks, and monitoring medication.

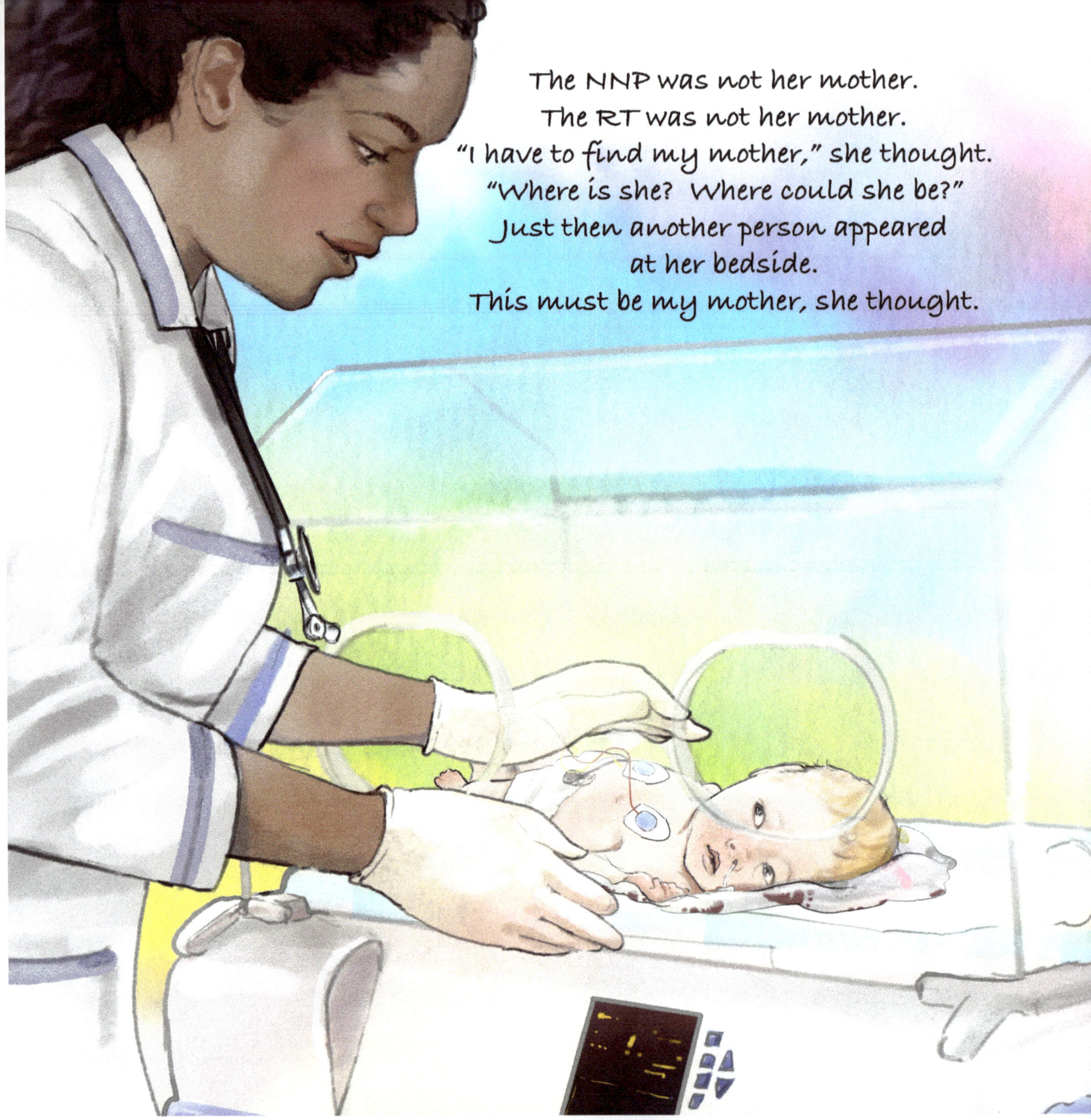
The NNP was not her mother.
The RT was not her mother.
"I have to find my mother," she thought.
"Where is she? Where could she be?"
Just then another person appeared
at her bedside.
This must be my mother, she thought.

"Are you my mother?" asked the baby.

"No, sweet pea, I am a Registered Nurse",
said the RN.

An RN (**Registered Nurse**) will be assigned to your baby around the clock, 7 days a week.

The RN works closely with you and the NNP / Neo to plan your baby's care.

The RN will be monitoring your baby closely, administering any medications your baby may need and providing all cares including feeding and diaper changes.

The NICU RN offers comfort and support to premature and ill newborns and their parents.

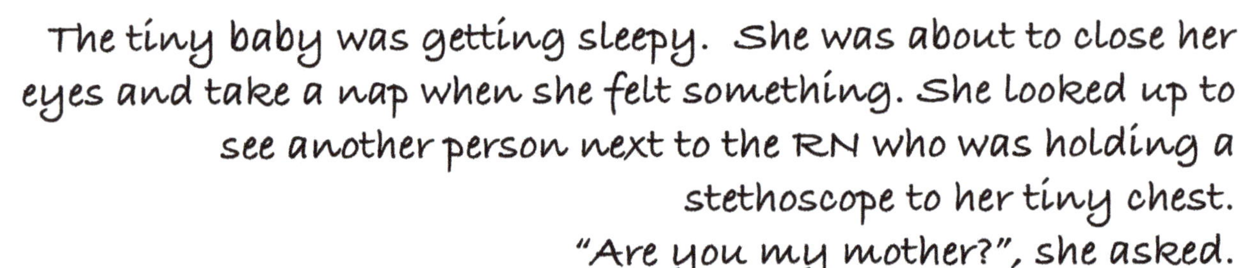

The tiny baby was getting sleepy. She was about to close her eyes and take a nap when she felt something. She looked up to see another person next to the RN who was holding a stethoscope to her tiny chest.
"Are you my mother?", she asked.
"I am not your mother,"
said the neonatologist.
"I am a neonatologist."

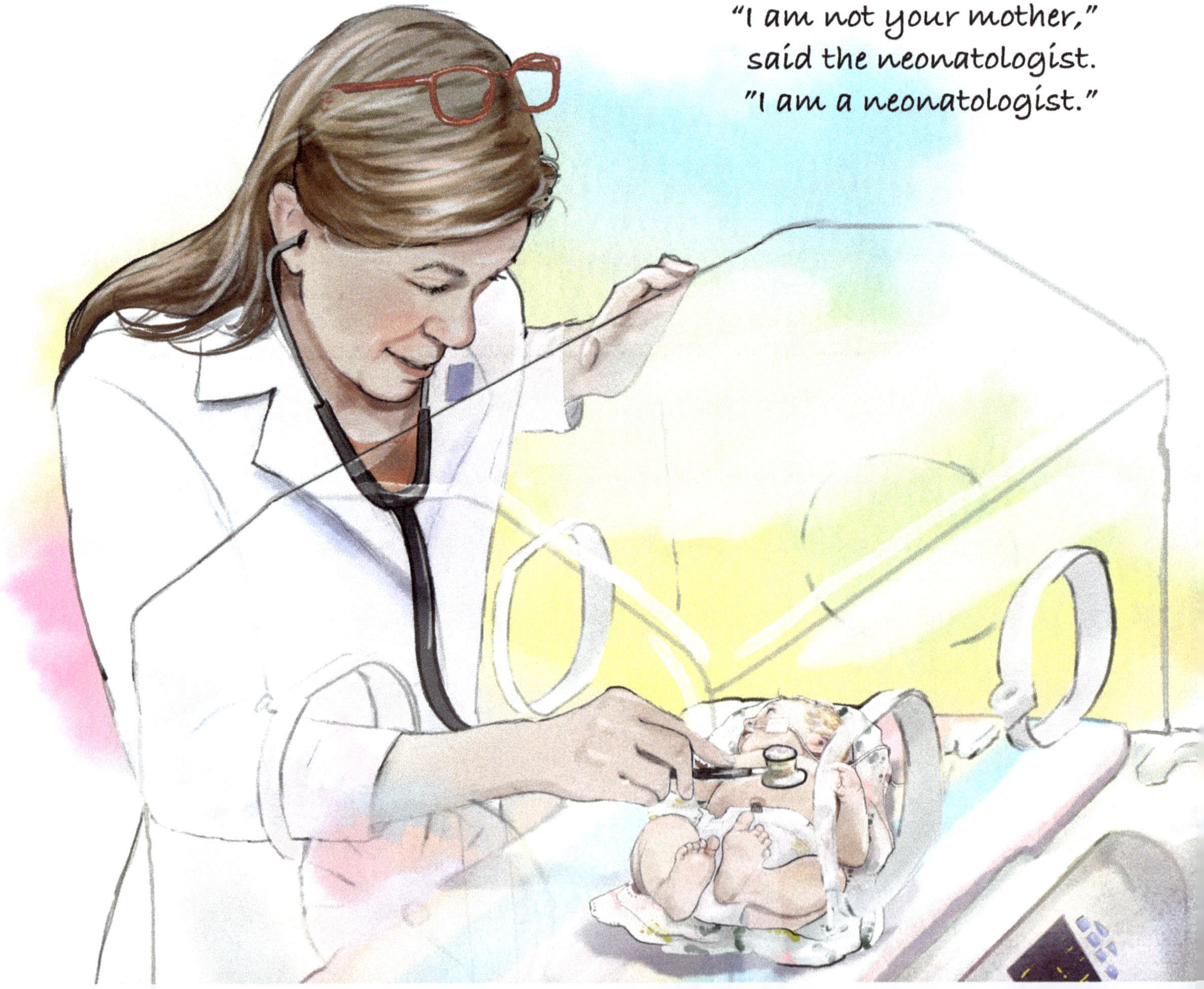

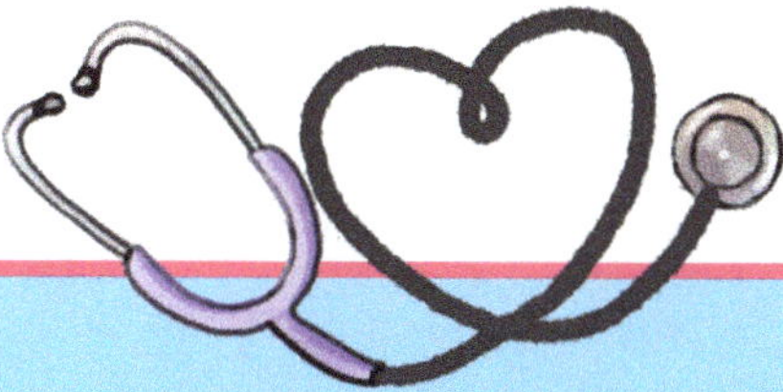

A **neonatologist** (Neo) is a physician with specialized training in caring for the most complex and high risk newborns, often premature infants or those in need of surgery.

Neonatologists use equipment that is designed specifically for the tiniest patients. They ensure that critically ill newborns receive the proper nutrition for healing and growth and prescribe any medication that your baby needs.

They will oversee your baby's care and will examine them daily.

The NNP was not her mother.
The RT and the RN were not her mother.
And the neonatologist was not her mother.
She decided to close her little eyes and rest.

Maybe she didn't have a mother.

But she knew she did. She did have a mother!

Just then, a person with a soft voice opened the door
of her isolette.

She turned her little face towards this new person and asked,

"Are you my mother?"

"No," laughing softly, replied the Physical Therapist.
"I am your physical therapist."

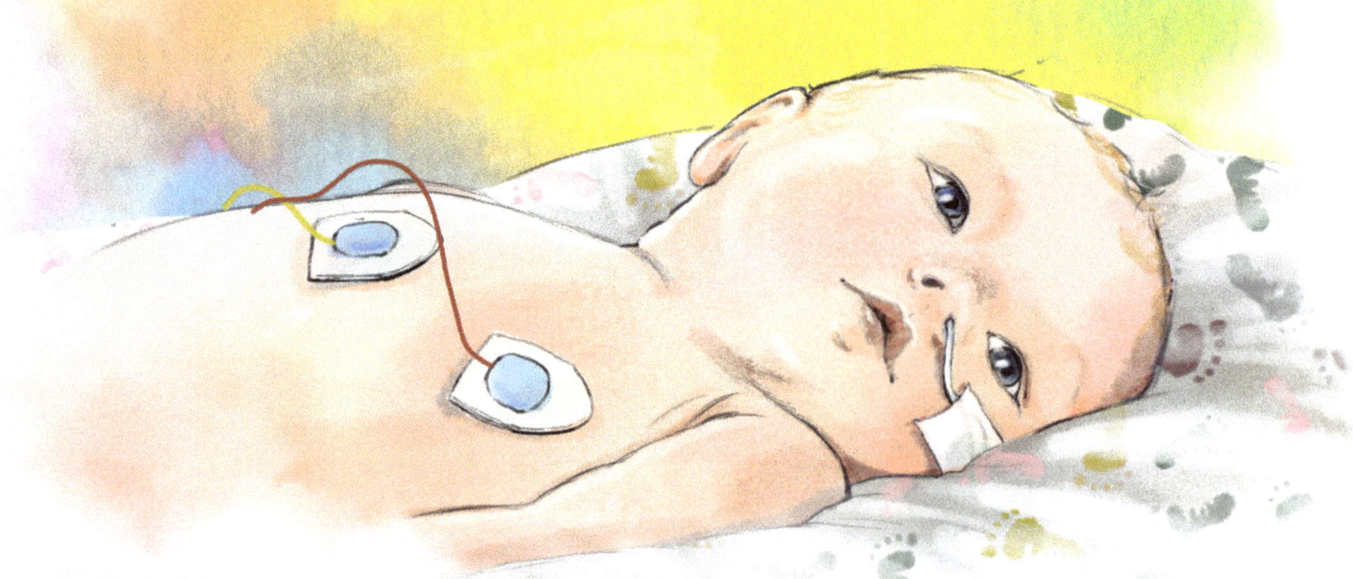

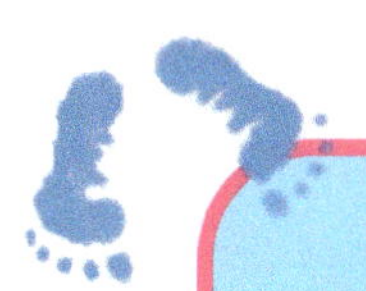

PTs (**Physical Therapists**) in the NICU have a thorough understanding of preterm and infant development and behavior. They will evaluate your baby's muscle tone, movement and sensory responses and implement therapies. They will also offer suggestions to you as a parent to support your baby's development and help you understand your baby's behaviors.

OTs (**Occupational Therapists**) strive to create a healing sensory environment for premature infants to grow and develop. Using the sensory system, the infant interprets the information around them through touch, smell, taste, sound and sight. An OT will help you assess and protect the development of your baby's sensory system. They may show you how to provide a quiet and dim environment for your baby while you participate in cares such as diaper changes, repositioning, holding and bathing. Positioning infants appropriately can help reduce head molding and decrease pressure in order to support good skin integrity. In addition, by using developmental positioners that are created specifically for tiny babies, both the PT and OT will demonstrate how to "nest" your baby to feel more secure. These containment positions mimic the womb by limiting movement and allow them to push against something for muscle development. Once your baby is stable, a PT and/or OT will typically work with your baby 2-3 times / week.

An SLP (**Speech Language Pathologist**) may do a pre-feeding readiness assessment to determine if your baby is ready to begin to breast or bottle feed. They will help you look for feeding cues and teach you how to feed your baby safely, including how to identify stress cues and signs of swallowing difficulties.

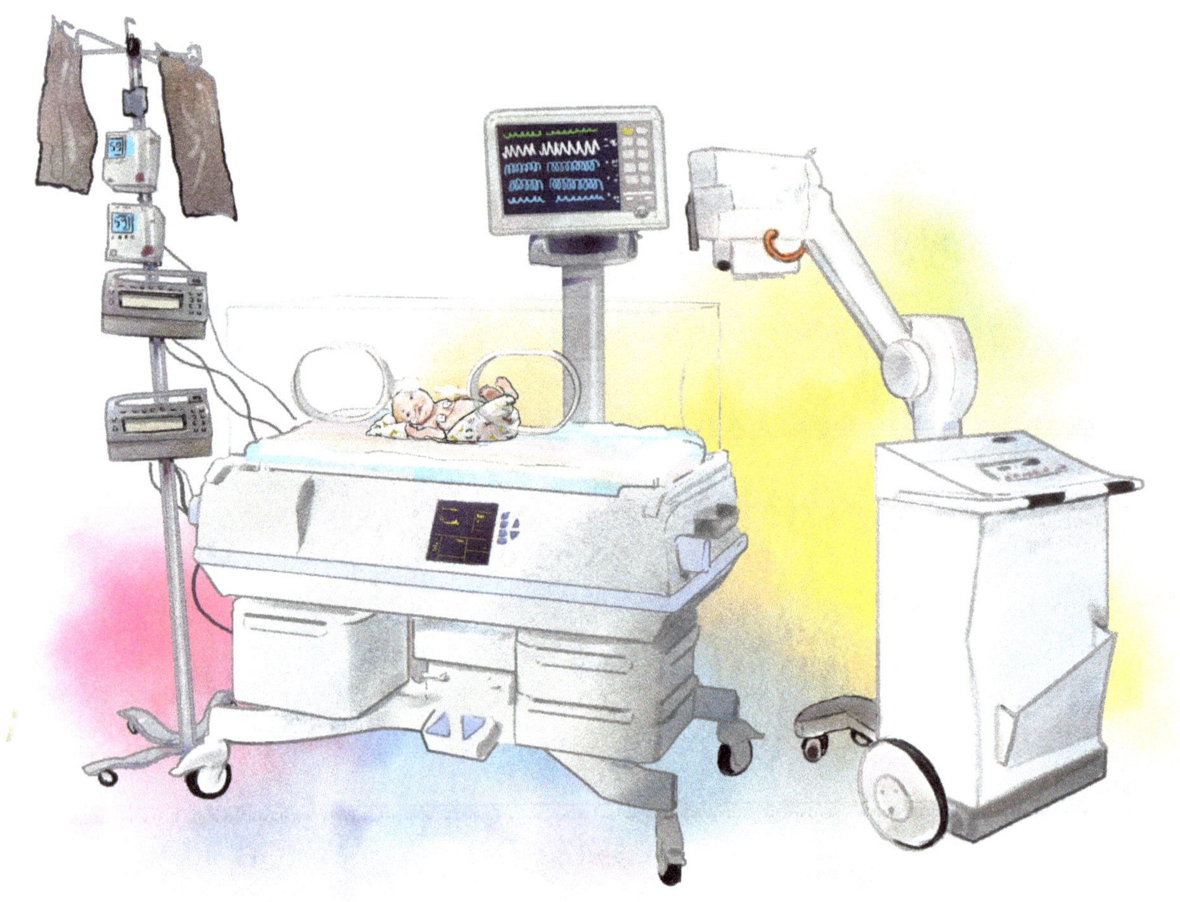

The little baby began to worry. She looked outside
of her isolette and saw a monitor with colorful
lines and numbers on it.
"There she is!", she thought, "could that be my mother?"
Suddenly, an xray machine was wheeled in.
Could that Big Thing be her mother?
"Mother! Here I am, mother!" she cried.
"Where am I? I want to go home! I want my mother!"

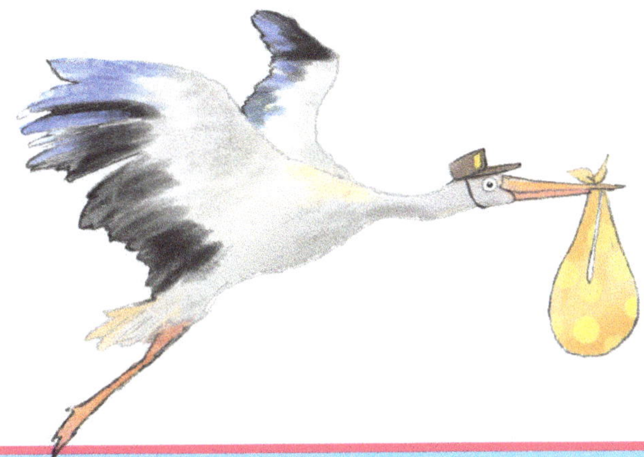

During your baby's NICU stay, depending on the level of care your baby needs, there may be several types of medical equipment connected to your baby.

The cardiopulmonary monitor will be measuring your baby's heart rate, breathing rates, and pulse oximetry (how much oxygen is in your baby's blood).

Your baby may require some type of ventilator to assist with breathing.

And the majority of babies will require a feeding tube for at least part of their stay. In addition, your baby may have some procedures done at the bedside including xrays, an echocardiogram or head ultrasound.

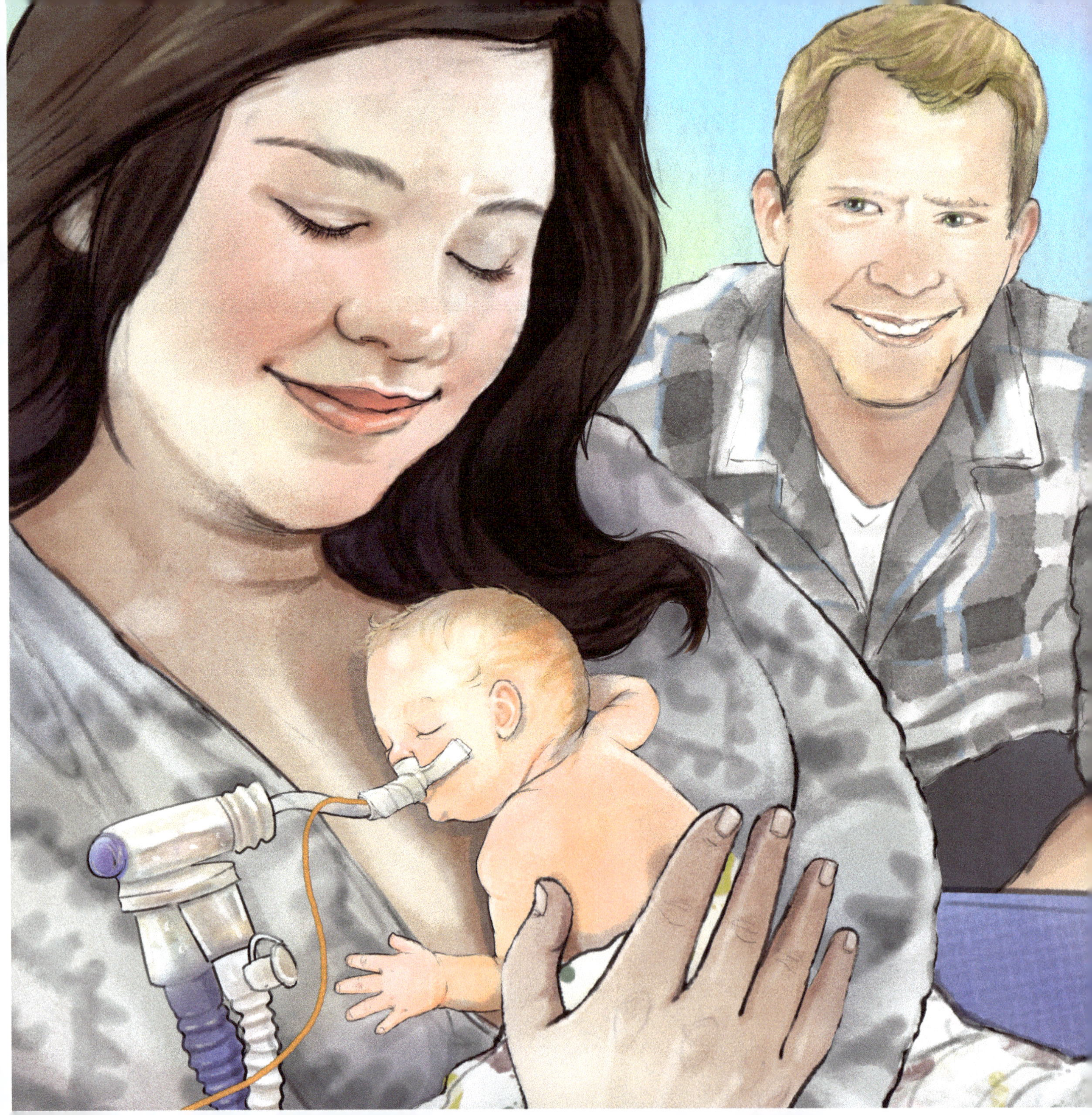

Just then, something happened.
The isolette door was lowered
and she was being carefully lifted out
and placed on her mother's chest…
The baby was home!
"Do you know who I am?" she said to her baby.
"Yes! I know who you are."

"You are not an NNP.
You are not an RT.
You are not an RN.
You are not a neonatologist.
You are not a PT,
or an OT,
or a speech pathologist, or a Big Thing."

"YOU ARE MY MOTHER!"

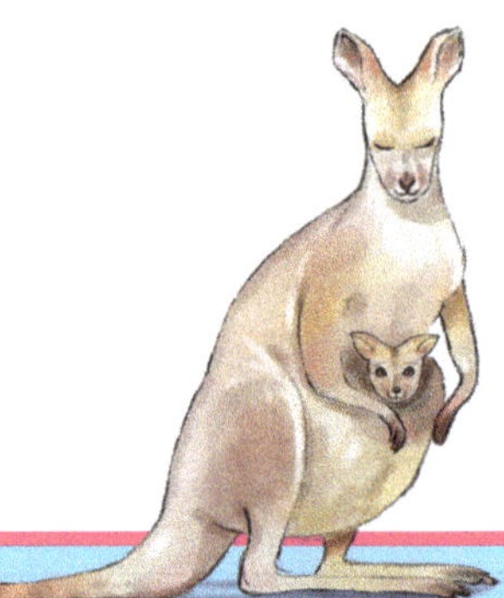

Parents are also very important members of the healthcare team! Ways you can contribute include being in regular communication with staff members and assisting with your baby's cares at touch times, (providing containment, taking baby's temperature, changing baby's diaper, and offering a pacifier).

You will bond with your baby through touching, feeding, and spending skin-to-skin (kangaroo care) time with your baby. Your baby will learn your smell and begin to recognize you.

Kangaroo care involves holding your baby skin-to-skin on your bare chest. There are many positive benefits of providing kangaroo care. These include improved oxygenation, helping your baby to stay warm, gain weight, sleep better, stabilize heart rate and respiratory rate, and help with growth and development of brain function.

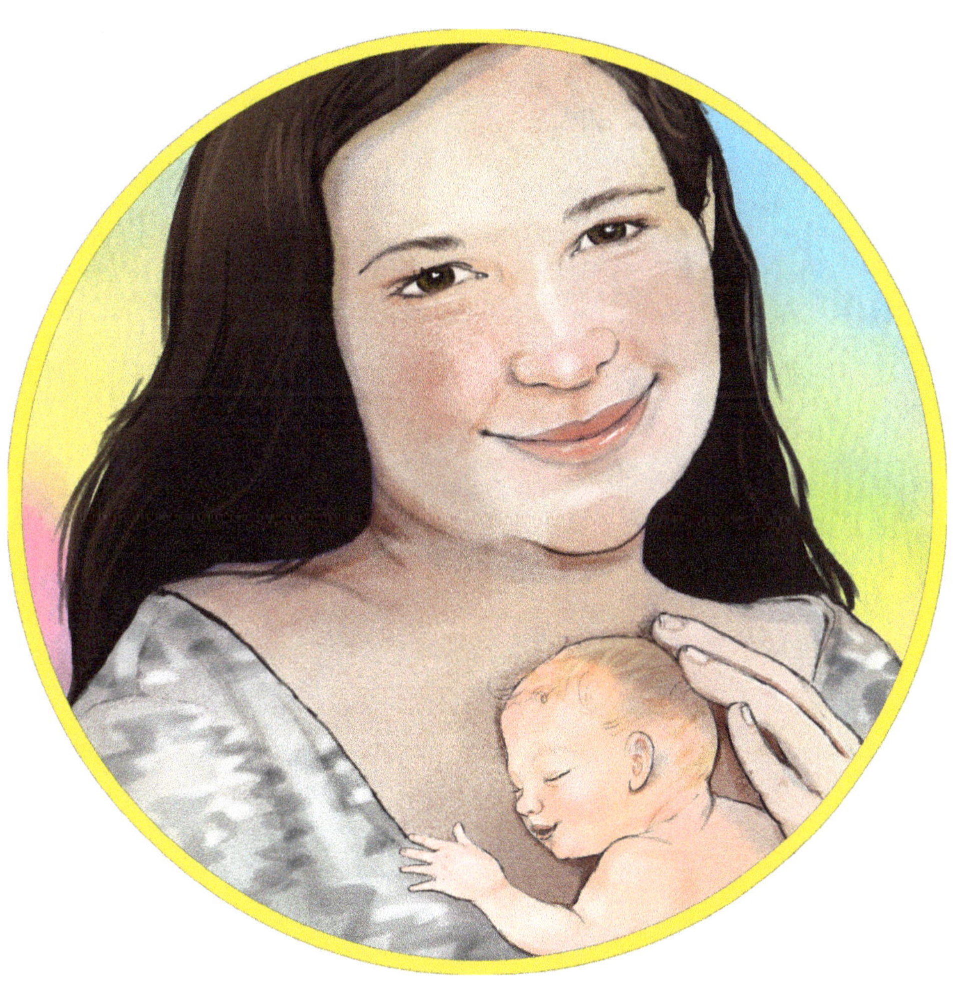

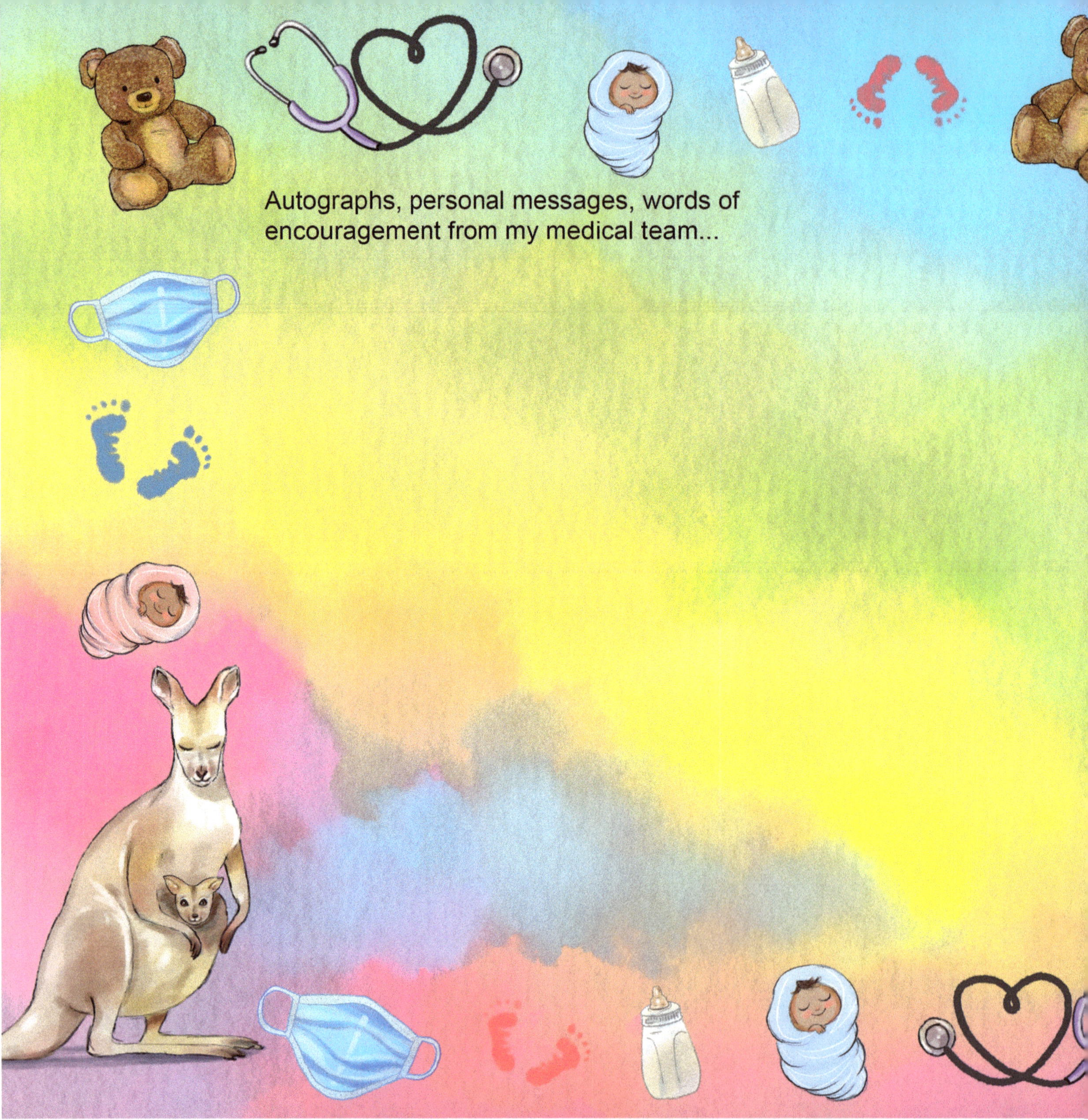

Autographs, personal messages, words of encouragement from my medical team...

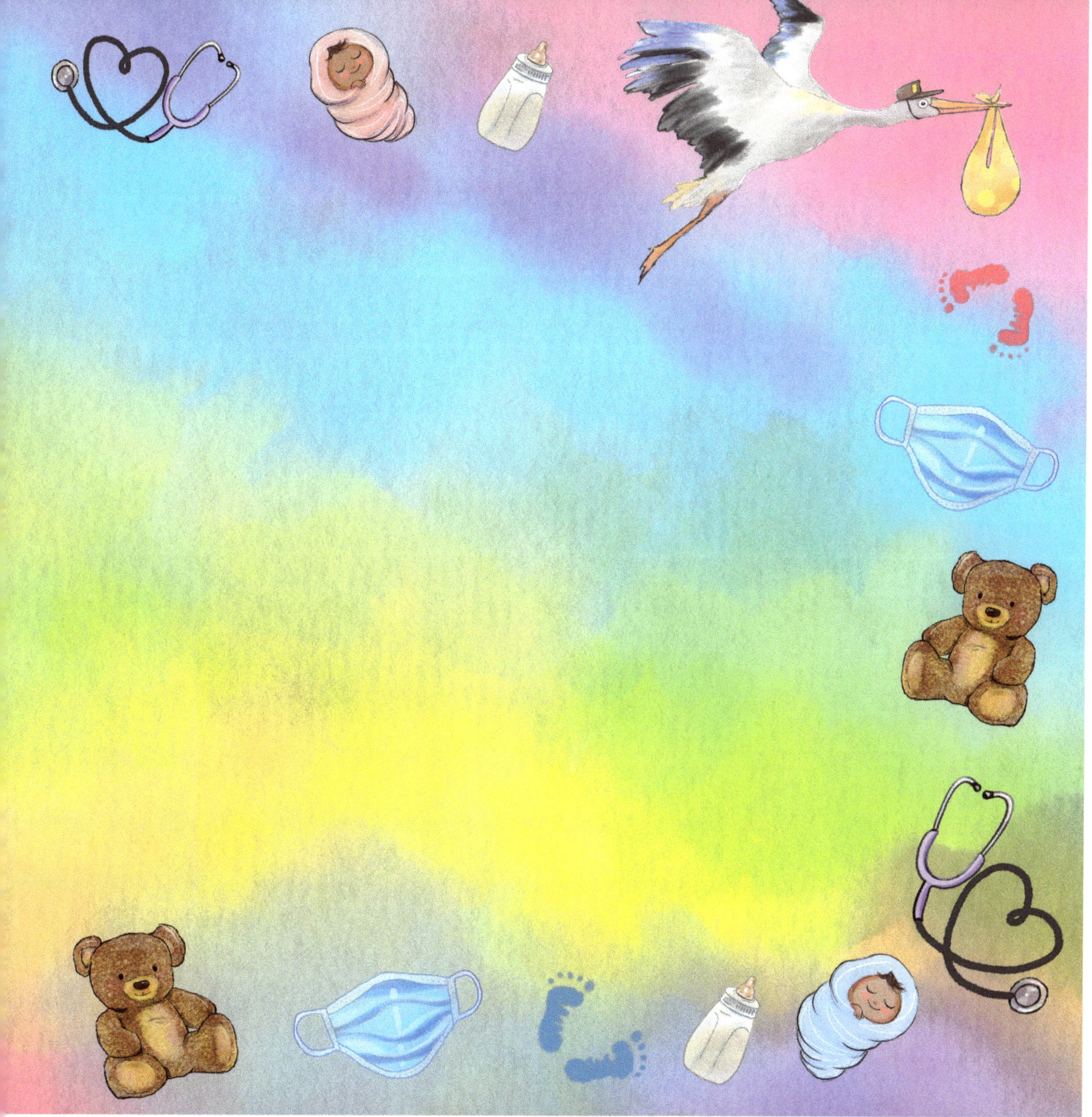

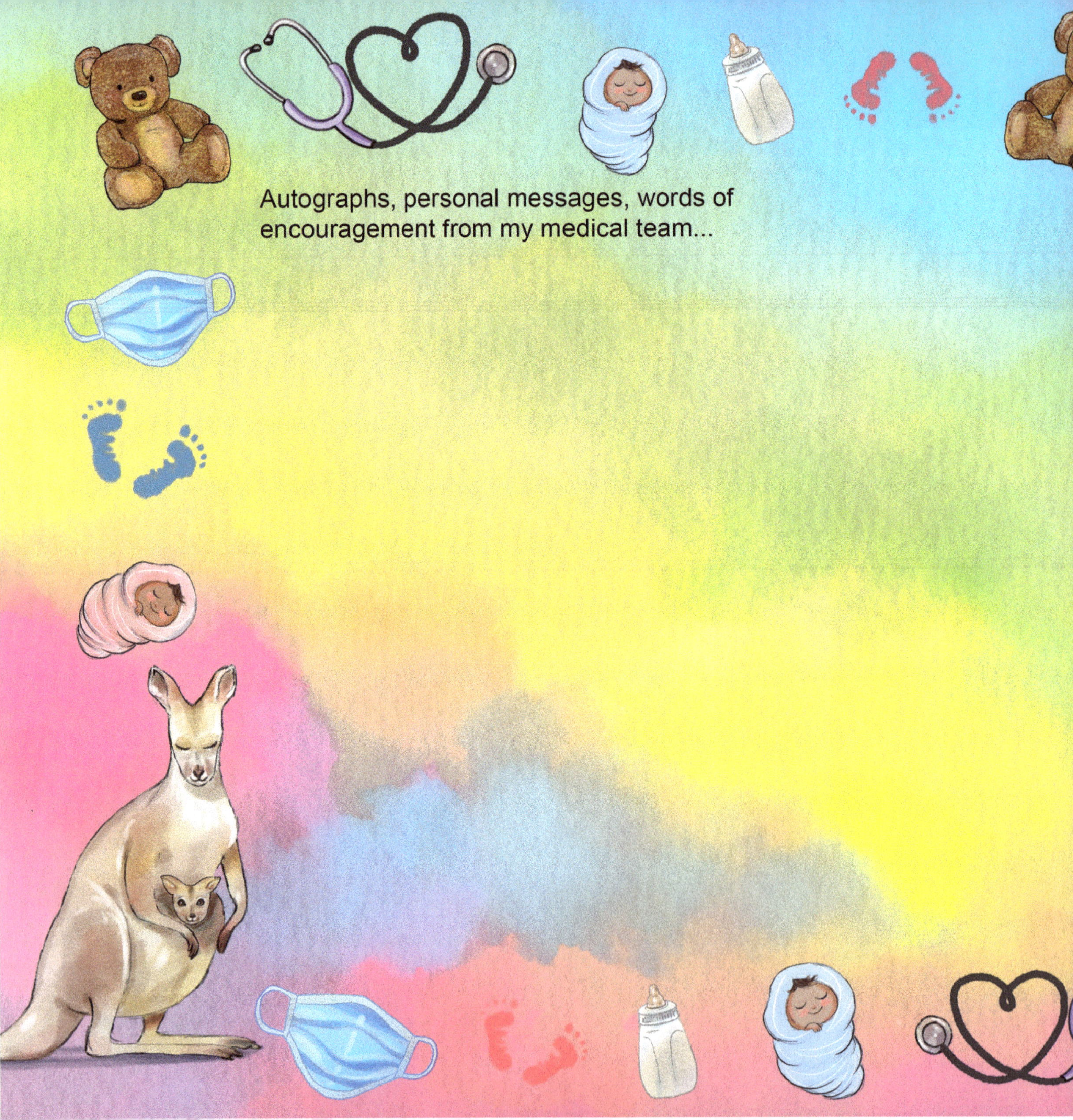

Autographs, personal messages, words of
encouragement from my medical team...

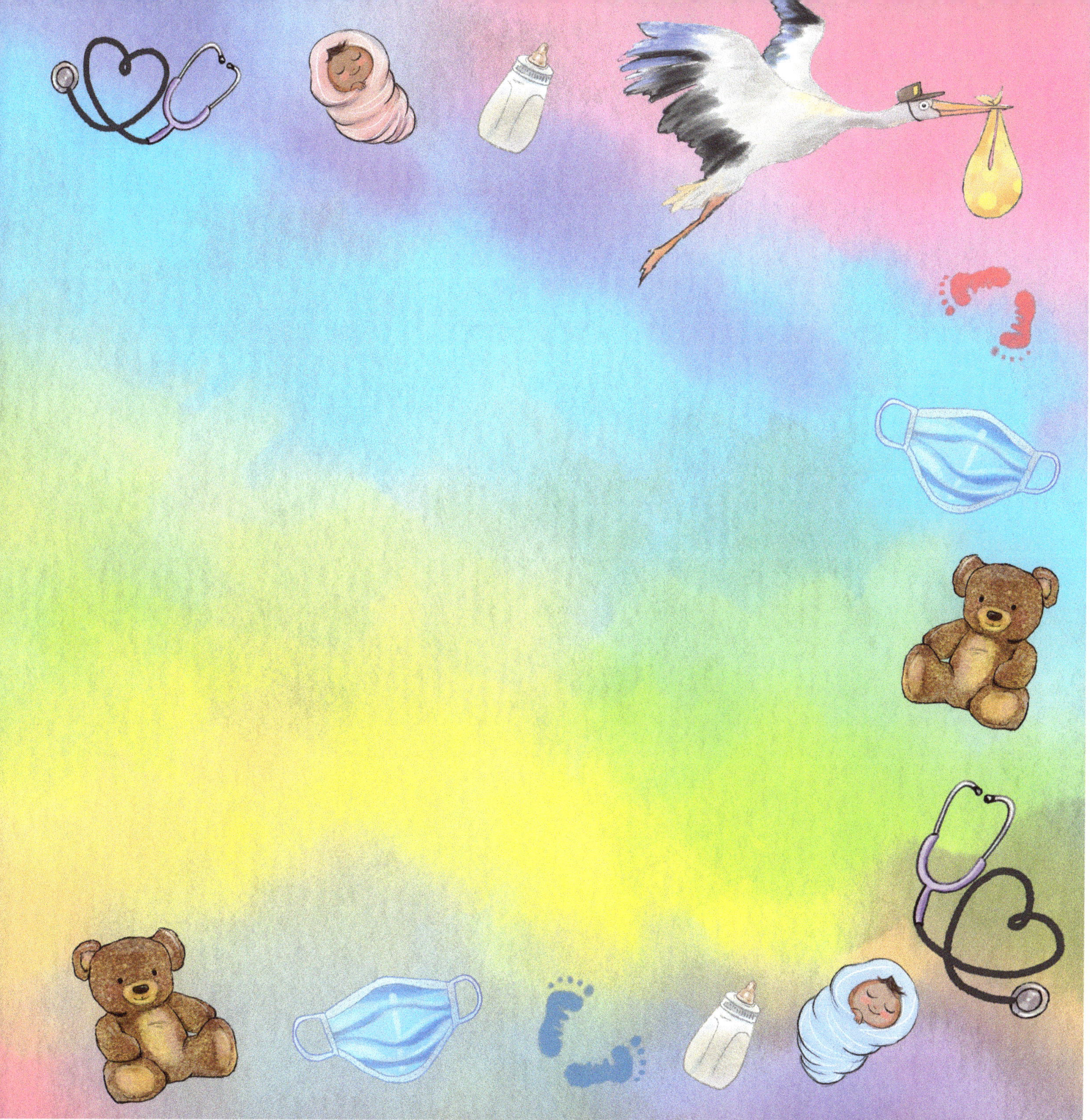

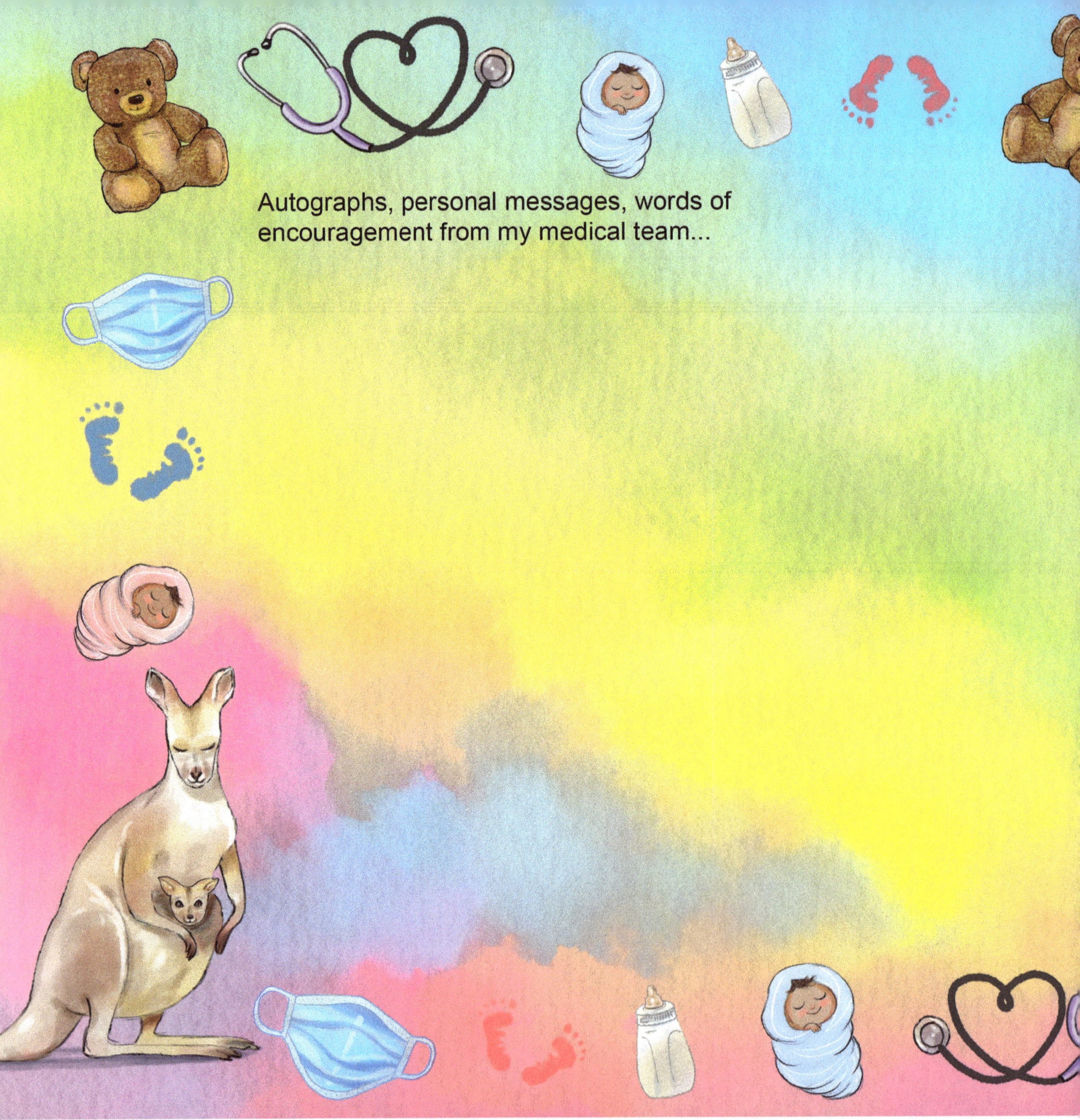

Autographs, personal messages, words of
encouragement from my medical team...